VEGAN DIABETIC KIDNEY DIET MEAL PLAN

Delicious and Nutritious Recipes for a Healthy Life

Dr Lily Morgan

COPYRIGHT PAGE

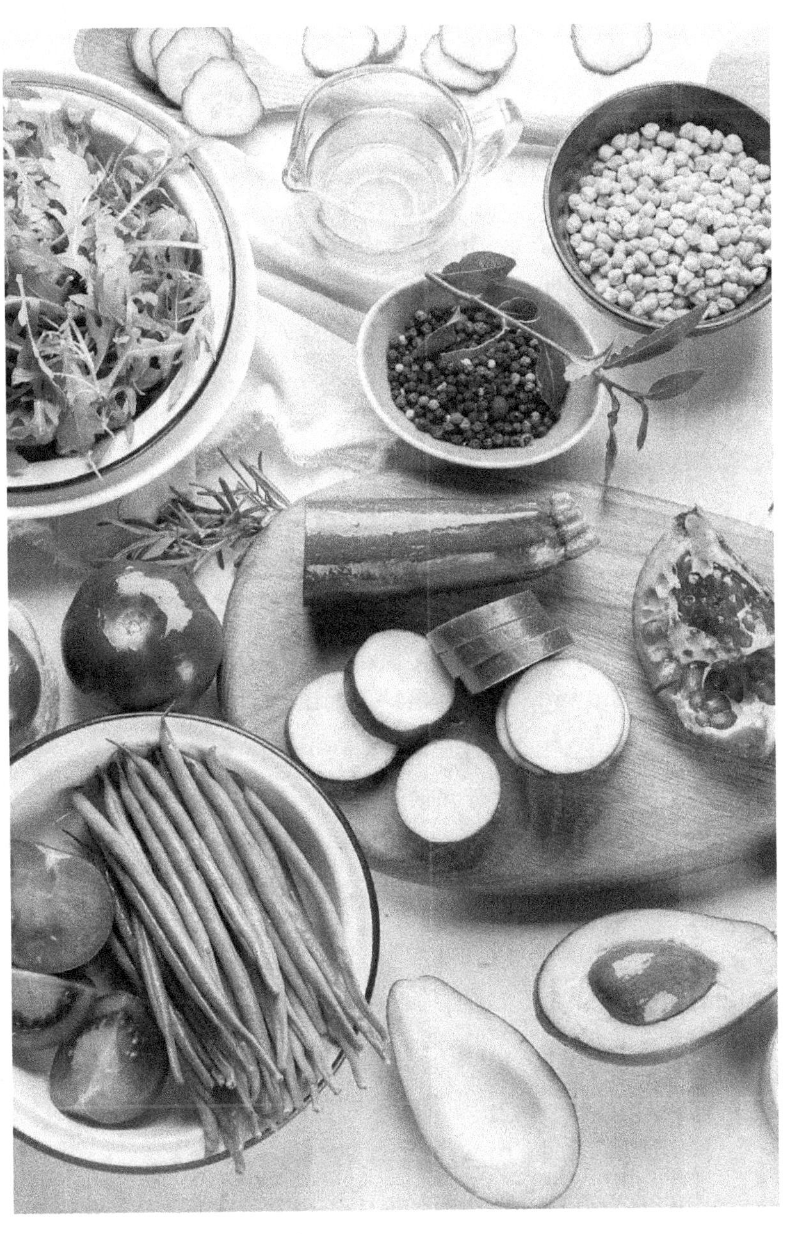

TABLE OF CONTENTS

Chapter 5: Snacks and Appetizers

INTRODUCTION

Diabetic Kidney Disease (DKD) is a chronic complication of diabetes that affects the kidneys' ability to filter waste and excess fluids from the bloodstream. It is a serious and potentially debilitating condition that requires careful management. This article aims to provide a genuine understanding of DKD and shed light on the remarkable benefits that a vegan diet can offer in its management.

What is Diabetic Kidney Disease (DKD)?

Diabetic Kidney Disease, also known as diabetic nephropathy, is a progressive kidney condition that arises as a result of longstanding diabetes. When blood sugar levels are consistently elevated, it can lead to damage in the small blood vessels within the kidneys. Over time, this damage impairs the kidneys' ability to filter waste and excess fluids, leading to a buildup of toxins in the body.

Common symptoms of DKD include:

1. Proteinuria: The presence of excess protein in the urine.
2. Edema: Swelling, particularly in the legs and ankles.
3. Hypertension: High blood pressure is a common complication of DKD.
4. Fatigue: Due to anemia and toxin buildup.
5. Reduced urine output: Kidneys may lose their ability to filter properly.

It's crucial to note that DKD often develops silently, with no noticeable symptoms in its early stages. Regular monitoring of blood glucose and kidney function is vital for early detection.

The Role of a Vegan Diet

Now, let's delve into the promising benefits of adopting a vegan diet for individuals with DKD:

Blood Sugar Control: A vegan diet primarily composed of plant-based foods such as fruits, vegetables, whole grains, and legumes can help stabilize blood sugar levels. These foods have a lower glycemic index, reducing the risk of blood sugar spikes.

Reduced Protein Intake: Managing protein intake is essential for DKD patients, as excessive protein can strain the kidneys. A vegan diet naturally reduces animal protein consumption, which can be beneficial for kidney health.

Lower Blood Pressure: Plant-based diets are often associated with lower blood pressure due to their reduced sodium content and high potassium levels. This can be especially advantageous for individuals with DKD, as hypertension is a common complication.

Kidney-Friendly Nutrients: Vegan diets provide ample vitamins, minerals, and antioxidants that support overall health and may reduce inflammation and oxidative stress in the kidneys.

Weight Management: Many people with diabetes struggle with weight management. A vegan diet, when balanced and well-planned, can assist in weight loss or maintenance, which is beneficial for diabetes and kidney health.

Reduced Risk of Heart Disease: Heart disease is a significant concern for DKD patients. Vegan diets are linked to a lower risk of heart disease, further enhancing overall well-being.

In summary, understanding Diabetic Kidney Disease is essential for early detection and management. Embracing a vegan diet, rich in plant-based foods, can offer a multitude of benefits for individuals with DKD, from better blood sugar control to improved kidney and heart health. However, it's crucial to consult with a healthcare professional and a registered dietitian before making significant dietary changes, as individual needs may vary.

Chapter 1: 30-Day Meal Plan

Week 1:

Day 1:

- Breakfast: Almond Butter and Banana Overnight Oats
- Lunch: Lentil and Vegetable Soup
- Dinner: Vegan Lentil Shepherd's Pie
- Snack: Guacamole with Veggie Sticks
- Dessert: Vegan Chocolate Avocado Mousse

Day 2:

- Breakfast: Spinach and Mushroom Vegan Quiche
- Lunch: Quinoa and Black Bean Salad
- Dinner: Zucchini Noodles with Pesto
- Snack: Vegan Spinach and Artichoke Dip
- Dessert: Vegan Blueberry Crisp

Day 3:

- Breakfast: Chia Seed Breakfast Pudding
- Lunch: Vegan Chickpea Salad

- Dinner: Butternut Squash Risotto
- Snack: Roasted Chickpeas
- Dessert: Vegan Banana Ice Cream

Day 4:

- Breakfast: Avocado Toast with a Twist
- Lunch: Stuffed Bell Peppers with Brown Rice
- Dinner: Vegan Chili
- Snack: Vegan Salsa and Tortilla Chips
- Dessert: Almond and Raspberry Thumbprint Cookies

Day 5:

- Breakfast: Berry and Spinach Smoothie Bowl
- Lunch: Spinach and Mushroom Quesadillas
- Dinner: Vegan Stuffed Cabbage Rolls
- Snack: Hummus and Cucumber Slices
- Dessert: Vegan Rice Pudding

Day 6:

- Breakfast: Tofu Scramble with Veggies
- Lunch: Tomato and Basil Zucchini Noodles

- Dinner: Portobello Mushroom Steaks
- Snack: Vegan Caprese Skewers
- Dessert: Vegan Chocolate Chip Cookies

Day 7:

- Breakfast: Peanut Butter and Berry Smoothie
- Lunch: Vegan Sushi Rolls
- Dinner: Cauliflower and Chickpea Curry
- Snack: Edamame with Sea Salt
- Dessert: Vegan Apple Crumble

Week 2:

Day 8:

- Breakfast: Sweet Potato Hash with Black Beans
- Lunch: Thai-Inspired Tofu Salad
- Dinner: Vegan Jambalaya
- Snack: Vegan Buffalo Cauliflower Bites
- Dessert: Vegan Lemon Bars

Day 9:

- Breakfast: Vegan Pancakes with Fresh Berries
- Lunch: Vegan Caesar Salad with Chickpea Croutons

- Dinner: Spinach and Artichoke Stuffed Peppers
- Snack: Stuffed Mushrooms
- Dessert: Vegan Chocolate Pots de Crème

Day 10:

- Breakfast: Green Breakfast Smoothie
- Lunch: Mediterranean Hummus Wrap
- Dinner: Vegan Pad Thai
- Snack: Vegan Spring Rolls
- Dessert: Vegan Pumpkin Pie

Day 11:

- Breakfast: Oatmeal with Cinnamon and Walnuts
- Lunch: Roasted Vegetable and Quinoa Bowl
- Dinner: Creamy Vegan Mushroom Pasta
- Snack: Vegan Bruschetta
- Dessert: Vegan Berry Sorbet

Day 12:

- Breakfast: Vegan Breakfast Burrito
- Lunch: Vegan Eggplant Parmesan
- Dinner: Vegan BBQ Tofu Skewers

- Snack: Vegan Popcorn with Nutritional Yeast
- Dessert: Vegan Peanut Butter Cups

Day 13:

- Breakfast: Blueberry Chia Jam on Whole-Grain Toast
- Lunch: Sweet Potato and Black Bean Tacos
- Dinner: Vegan Eggplant and Tomato Bake
- Snack: Vegan Sweet Potato Fries
- Dessert: Vegan Tiramisu

Day 14:

- Breakfast: Vegan Yogurt Parfait
- Lunch: Vegan Greek Salad
- Dinner: Vegan Spaghetti Carbonara
- Snack: Vegan Olive Tapenade
- Dessert: Vegan Coconut Macaroons

Week 3:

Day 15:

- Breakfast: Vegetable and Rice Congee
- Lunch: Curry Chickpea Salad

- Dinner: Quinoa-Stuffed Acorn Squash
- Snack: Vegan Nachos with Cashew Cheese
- Dessert: Vegan Carrot Cake

Day 16:

- Breakfast: Almond Butter and Banana Overnight Oats
- Lunch: Lentil and Vegetable Soup
- Dinner: Vegan Lentil Shepherd's Pie
- Snack: Guacamole with Veggie Sticks
- Dessert: Vegan Chocolate Avocado Mousse

Day 17:

- Breakfast: Spinach and Mushroom Vegan Quiche
- Lunch: Quinoa and Black Bean Salad
- Dinner: Zucchini Noodles with Pesto
- Snack: Vegan Spinach and Artichoke Dip
- Dessert: Vegan Blueberry Crisp

Day 18:

- Breakfast: Chia Seed Breakfast Pudding
- Lunch: Vegan Chickpea Salad

- Dinner: Butternut Squash Risotto
- Snack: Roasted Chickpeas
- Dessert: Vegan Banana Ice Cream

Day 19:

- Breakfast: Avocado Toast with a Twist
- Lunch: Stuffed Bell Peppers with Brown Rice
- Dinner: Vegan Chili
- Snack: Vegan Salsa and Tortilla Chips
- Dessert: Almond and Raspberry Thumbprint Cookies

Day 20:

- Breakfast: Berry and Spinach Smoothie Bowl
- Lunch: Spinach and Mushroom Quesadillas
- Dinner: Vegan Stuffed Cabbage Rolls
- Snack: Hummus and Cucumber Slices
- Dessert: Vegan Rice Pudding

Day 21:

- Breakfast: Tofu Scramble with Veggies
- Lunch: Tomato and Basil Zucchini Noodles

- Dinner: Portobello Mushroom Steaks
- Snack: Vegan Caprese Skewers
- Dessert: Vegan Chocolate Chip Cookies

Week 4:

Day 22:

- Breakfast: Peanut Butter and Berry Smoothie
- Lunch: Vegan Sushi Rolls
- Dinner: Cauliflower and Chickpea Curry
- Snack: Edamame with Sea Salt
- Dessert: Vegan Apple Crumble

Day 23:

- Breakfast: Sweet Potato Hash with Black Beans
- Lunch: Thai-Inspired Tofu Salad
- Dinner: Vegan Jambalaya
- Snack: Vegan Buffalo Cauliflower Bites
- Dessert: Vegan Lemon Bars

Day 24:

- Breakfast: Vegan Pancakes with Fresh Berries
- Lunch: Vegan Caesar Salad with Chickpea Croutons

- Dinner: Spinach and Artichoke Stuffed Peppers
- Snack: Stuffed Mushrooms
- Dessert: Vegan Chocolate Pots de Crème

Day 25:

- Breakfast: Green Breakfast Smoothie
- Lunch: Mediterranean Hummus Wrap
- Dinner: Vegan Pad Thai
- Snack: Vegan Spring Rolls
- Dessert: Vegan Pumpkin Pie

Day 26:

- Breakfast: Oatmeal with Cinnamon and Walnuts
- Lunch: Roasted Vegetable and Quinoa Bowl
- Dinner: Creamy Vegan Mushroom Pasta
- Snack: Vegan Bruschetta
- Dessert: Vegan Berry Sorbet

Day 27:

- Breakfast: Vegan Breakfast Burrito
- Lunch: Vegan Eggplant Parmesan
- Dinner: Vegan BBQ Tofu Skewers

- Snack: Vegan Popcorn with Nutritional Yeast
- Dessert: Vegan Peanut Butter Cups

Day 28:

- Breakfast: Blueberry Chia Jam on Whole-Grain Toast
- Lunch: Sweet Potato and Black Bean Tacos
- Dinner: Vegan Eggplant and Tomato Bake
- Snack: Vegan Sweet Potato Fries
- Dessert: Vegan Tiramisu

Day 29:

- Breakfast: Vegan Yogurt Parfait
- Lunch: Vegan Greek Salad
- Dinner: Vegan Spaghetti Carbonara
- Snack: Vegan Olive Tapenade
- Dessert: Vegan Coconut Macaroons

Day 30:

- Breakfast: Vegetable and Rice Congee
- Lunch: Curry Chickpea Salad
- Dinner: Quinoa-Stuffed Acorn Squash

- Snack: Vegan Nachos with Cashew Cheese
- Dessert: Vegan Carrot Cake

This completes the 30-day meal plan with a diverse selection of recipes. Feel free to adjust portion sizes and ingredients to suit your dietary preferences and needs. Enjoy your journey to better health!

Chapter 2: Breakfast Recipes

Breakfast is the foundation of your day, providing you with the energy and nutrients needed to start your morning right. In this chapter, we've curated a delightful collection of breakfast recipes that are not only delicious but also tailored to keep your blood sugar in check.

Almond Butter and Banana Overnight Oats

Ingredients:

- 1/2 cup rolled oats
- 1 cup almond milk
- 1 tablespoon almond butter
- 1 ripe banana, mashed
- 1 teaspoon honey (optional)
- Sliced almonds for garnish

Instructions:

1. In a jar, combine oats and almond milk.

2. Stir in almond butter, mashed banana, and honey (if desired).

3. Seal the jar and refrigerate overnight.

4. Top with sliced almonds before serving.

Spinach and Mushroom Vegan Quiche

Ingredients:

- 1 pre-made vegan pie crust
- 1 cup spinach, chopped
- 1 cup mushrooms, sliced
- 1/2 cup cherry tomatoes, halved
- 1 cup tofu, crumbled
- 1/4 cup nutritional yeast
- 1/2 teaspoon turmeric
- Salt and pepper to taste

Instructions:

1. Preheat your oven to 375°F (190°C).

2. Sauté spinach, mushrooms, and cherry tomatoes until tender.

3. In a bowl, mix crumbled tofu, nutritional yeast, turmeric, salt, and pepper.

4. Transfer the sautéed veggies to the pie crust, then pour the tofu mixture over them.

5. Bake for 30-35 minutes, or until the quiche is set.

Chia Seed Breakfast Pudding

Ingredients:

- 3 tablespoons chia seeds
- 1 cup almond milk
- 1/2 teaspoon vanilla extract
- Fresh berries for topping

Instructions:

1. Mix chia seeds, almond milk, and vanilla extract in a jar.

2. Seal the jar and refrigerate for at least 2 hours (or overnight).

3. Top with fresh berries before enjoying.

Avocado Toast with a Twist

Ingredients:

- 2 slices whole-grain bread
- 1 ripe avocado, mashed
- Cherry tomatoes, sliced
- Red pepper flakes
- Lemon juice
- Salt and pepper to taste

Instructions:

1. Toast the bread until golden brown.
2. Spread mashed avocado on the toast.
3. Top with sliced cherry tomatoes.
4. Drizzle with lemon juice and sprinkle red pepper flakes, salt, and pepper.

Berry and Spinach Smoothie Bowl

Ingredients:

- 1 cup fresh spinach
- 1/2 cup mixed berries (strawberries, blueberries, raspberries)

- 1/2 banana
- 1/2 cup almond milk
- Toppings: sliced bananas, granola, chia seeds

Instructions:

1. Blend spinach, mixed berries, banana, and almond milk until smooth.
2. Pour into a bowl and add your favorite toppings.

Tofu Scramble with Veggies

Ingredients:

- 1/2 block of firm tofu, crumbled
- 1/2 cup bell peppers, diced
- 1/2 cup onions, diced
- 1/2 cup spinach, chopped
- 1 clove garlic, minced
- 1/2 teaspoon turmeric
- Salt and pepper to taste

Instructions:

1. Sauté onions, bell peppers, and garlic until softened.
2. Add crumbled tofu, turmeric, salt, and pepper.

3. Cook until tofu is heated through.

4. Stir in chopped spinach until wilted.

Peanut Butter and Berry Smoothie

Ingredients:

- 1 cup mixed berries (strawberries, blueberries, raspberries)
- 2 tablespoons peanut butter
- 1 cup almond milk
- 1 ripe banana
- 1 tablespoon chia seeds

Instructions:

1. Blend mixed berries, peanut butter, almond milk, and banana until smooth.

2. Sprinkle chia seeds on top before serving.

Sweet Potato Hash with Black Beans

Ingredients:

- 2 sweet potatoes, diced

- 1 can black beans, drained and rinsed
- 1 red bell pepper, diced
- 1 onion, diced
- 1 teaspoon paprika
- Salt and pepper to taste

Instructions:

1. Heat olive oil in a pan and add diced sweet potatoes.
2. Sauté until potatoes are tender.
3. Add diced onion and red bell pepper.
4. Stir in black beans, paprika, salt, and pepper.
5. Cook until heated through.

Vegan Pancakes with Fresh Berries

Ingredients:

- 1 cup whole wheat flour
- 1 tablespoon baking powder
- 1 tablespoon maple syrup
- 1 cup almond milk
- Fresh berries for topping

Instructions:

1. Mix whole wheat flour and baking powder in a bowl.

2. Add maple syrup and almond milk, stir until smooth.

3. Pour the batter onto a hot griddle and cook until bubbles form.

4. Flip and cook until golden brown.

5. Serve with fresh berries on top.

Green Breakfast Smoothie

Ingredients:

- 2 cups kale leaves, stems removed

- 1 cup pineapple chunks

- 1/2 banana

- 1 cup coconut water

- 1 tablespoon flax seeds

Instructions:

1. Blend kale, pineapple, banana, coconut water, and flax seeds until smooth.

2. Enjoy the green goodness!

Oatmeal with Cinnamon and Walnuts

Ingredients:

- 1/2 cup rolled oats
- 1 cup water or almond milk
- 1/2 teaspoon ground cinnamon
- 1/4 cup chopped walnuts
- Sliced bananas for garnish

Instructions:

1. Combine oats and water/almond milk in a pot.
2. Cook over low heat, stirring occasionally, until creamy.
3. Stir in ground cinnamon and chopped walnuts.
4. Serve with sliced bananas on top.

Vegan Breakfast Burrito

Ingredients:

- 1 whole-grain tortilla
- 1/2 cup black beans, cooked and mashed
- 1/4 cup diced tomatoes

- 1/4 cup diced avocado

- Salsa for drizzling

- Fresh cilantro for garnish

Instructions:

1. Warm the tortilla.

2. Spread mashed black beans on the tortilla.

3. Add diced tomatoes and avocado.

4. Drizzle with salsa and garnish with fresh cilantro.

5. Roll up and enjoy.

Blueberry Chia Jam on Whole-Grain Toast

Ingredients:

- 1 cup blueberries

- 2 tablespoons chia seeds

- 1 tablespoon maple syrup

- Whole-grain toast

Instructions:

1. In a saucepan, heat blueberries and maple syrup until they start to break down.
2. Stir in chia seeds and cook until the jam thickens.
3. Spread the jam on whole-grain toast.

Vegan Yogurt Parfait

Ingredients:

- 1 cup dairy-free yogurt
- 1/2 cup granola
- Mixed berries
- Drizzle of agave syrup (optional)

Instructions:

1. Layer yogurt, granola, and mixed berries in a glass.
2. Repeat the layers.
3. Drizzle with agave syrup if desired.

Vegetable and Rice Congee

Ingredients:

- 1/2 cup white rice

- 4 cups vegetable broth
- 1 cup mixed vegetables (carrots, peas, corn)
- Soy sauce and sesame oil to taste
- Green onions for garnish

Instructions:

1. Rinse the rice and place it in a pot with vegetable broth.
2. Bring to a boil, then simmer until the rice is soft and creamy.
3. Stir in mixed vegetables, soy sauce, and sesame oil.
4. Simmer until vegetables are tender.
5. Garnish with chopped green onions.

Chapter 3: Lunch Recipes

In this chapter, we delve into a delightful array of vegan lunch recipes designed to tantalize your taste buds while keeping your health in mind. Whether you're seeking a refreshing salad, a hearty wrap, or a flavorful bowl, these recipes offer a wide range of flavors and textures to satisfy your midday cravings.

Lentil and Vegetable Soup

Ingredients:

- 1 cup dried green lentils
- 4 cups vegetable broth
- 1 onion, chopped
- 2 carrots, diced
- 2 celery stalks, sliced
- 2 cloves garlic, minced
- 1 can diced tomatoes
- 1 teaspoon cumin
- 1 teaspoon paprika
- Salt and pepper to taste

- Fresh parsley for garnish

Instructions:

1. Rinse lentils and set aside.

2. In a large pot, sauté onions, carrots, and celery until softened.

3. Add garlic, cumin, and paprika; cook for 1 minute.

4. Add lentils, vegetable broth, and diced tomatoes. Simmer for 30-40 minutes until lentils are tender.

5. Season with salt and pepper, garnish with fresh parsley, and serve.

Quinoa and Black Bean Salad

Ingredients:

- 1 cup quinoa, rinsed

- 2 cups water

- 1 can black beans, drained and rinsed

- 1 cup corn kernels (fresh or frozen)

- 1 red bell pepper, diced

- 1/4 cup red onion, finely chopped

- 1/4 cup fresh cilantro, chopped

- Juice of 2 limes

- 2 tablespoons olive oil
- Salt and pepper to taste

Instructions:

1. Cook quinoa in water according to package instructions, then let it cool.
2. In a large bowl, combine cooked quinoa, black beans, corn, bell pepper, red onion, and cilantro.
3. In a separate bowl, whisk together lime juice, olive oil, salt, and pepper.
4. Pour the dressing over the salad and toss well.
5. Chill in the refrigerator before serving.

Vegan Chickpea Salad

Ingredients:

- 2 cans chickpeas, drained and rinsed
- 1 cucumber, diced
- 1 red bell pepper, chopped
- 1/4 cup red onion, finely chopped
- 1/4 cup fresh parsley, chopped
- Juice of 1 lemon
- 2 tablespoons olive oil

- 1 teaspoon cumin

- Salt and pepper to taste

Instructions:

1. In a large bowl, combine chickpeas, cucumber, red bell pepper, red onion, and parsley.

2. In a separate bowl, whisk together lemon juice, olive oil, cumin, salt, and pepper.

3. Pour the dressing over the salad and toss to coat.

4. Let it sit for a few minutes to allow the flavors to meld before serving.

Stuffed Bell Peppers with Brown Rice

Ingredients:

- 4 bell peppers (any color)

- 1 cup brown rice, cooked

- 1 can black beans, drained and rinsed

- 1 cup corn kernels (fresh or frozen)

- 1/2 cup diced tomatoes

- 1/2 cup diced red onion

- 1/2 cup vegan cheese (optional)
- 1 teaspoon chili powder
- Salt and pepper to taste

Instructions:

1. Preheat the oven to 350°F (175°C).
2. Cut the tops off the bell peppers and remove the seeds and membranes.
3. In a bowl, combine cooked brown rice, black beans, corn, diced tomatoes, red onion, vegan cheese (if desired), chili powder, salt, and pepper.
4. Stuff each bell pepper with the mixture.
5. Place the stuffed peppers in a baking dish, cover with foil, and bake for 30 minutes.
6. Remove the foil and bake for an additional 15 minutes until peppers are tender.

Spinach and Mushroom Quesadillas

Ingredients:

- 4 large whole wheat tortillas
- 2 cups fresh spinach leaves
- 2 cups mushrooms, sliced

- 1 red onion, thinly sliced
- 1 cup vegan cheese, shredded
- Olive oil for cooking
- Salt and pepper to taste

Instructions:

1. In a skillet, heat olive oil over medium heat.
2. Add sliced mushrooms and red onion, sauté until softened.
3. Add fresh spinach and cook until wilted. Season with salt and pepper.
4. Place one tortilla in the skillet, sprinkle with vegan cheese, and add the mushroom-spinach mixture.
5. Top with another tortilla and press gently.
6. Cook until the tortilla is crispy and cheese is melted, then flip and cook the other side.
7. Repeat for the remaining quesadillas.
8. Cut into wedges and serve with salsa or guacamole.

Tomato and Basil Zucchini Noodles

Ingredients:

- 4 medium zucchinis, spiralized into noodles

- 2 cups cherry tomatoes, halved
- 2 cloves garlic, minced
- 1/4 cup fresh basil, chopped
- 2 tablespoons olive oil
- Salt and pepper to taste
- Vegan parmesan cheese (optional)

Instructions:

1. In a large skillet, heat olive oil over medium heat.

2. Add minced garlic and cherry tomatoes, sauté for a few minutes until tomatoes soften.

3. Add zucchini noodles and toss to combine. Cook for 2-3 minutes until heated through.

4. Season with salt and pepper, then stir in fresh basil.

5. Optional: Sprinkle with vegan parmesan cheese before serving.

Vegan Sushi Rolls

Ingredients:

- 4 nori sheets
- 2 cups sushi rice, cooked and seasoned with rice vinegar

- 1/2 cucumber, julienned
- 1/2 avocado, sliced
- 1/2 carrot, julienned
- 1/2 red bell pepper, julienned
- Soy sauce and pickled ginger for dipping

Instructions:

1. Place a bamboo sushi rolling mat on a clean surface.
2. Lay a sheet of plastic wrap on the mat, then place a nori sheet on top.
3. Wet your hands and spread a thin layer of sushi rice over the nori, leaving a small border at the top.
4. Arrange cucumber, avocado, carrot, and red bell pepper in the center.
5. Roll up the sushi using the bamboo mat, applying gentle pressure as you go.
6. Wet the top border of nori to seal the roll.
7. Slice the roll into bite-sized pieces and serve with soy sauce and pickled ginger.

Thai-Inspired Tofu Salad

Ingredients:

- 1 block extra-firm tofu, cubed
- 1 tablespoon soy sauce
- 2 cups mixed greens
- 1/2 cup shredded carrots
- 1/2 cup sliced cucumber
- 1/4 cup fresh cilantro leaves
- 1/4 cup chopped peanuts
- Lime wedges for garnish
- Thai peanut dressing

Instructions:

1. Marinate tofu cubes in soy sauce for 15 minutes.
2. Pan-fry or bake tofu until crispy and golden.
3. Assemble mixed greens, shredded carrots, sliced cucumber, and fresh cilantro in a bowl.
4. Top with crispy tofu and chopped peanuts.
5. Drizzle with Thai peanut dressing and garnish with lime wedges.

Vegan Caesar Salad with Chickpea Croutons

Ingredients:

- 4 cups romaine lettuce, chopped
- 1 cup cherry tomatoes, halved
- 1/4 cup vegan Caesar dressing
- 1/4 cup nutritional yeast (for "Parmesan")
-

Chickpea croutons:

- 1 can chickpeas, drained and rinsed
- 1 tablespoon olive oil
- 1 teaspoon garlic powder
- Salt and pepper to taste

Instructions:

1. Preheat oven to 400°F (200°C).
2. In a bowl, toss chickpeas with olive oil, garlic powder, salt, and pepper.
3. Spread chickpeas on a baking sheet and roast for 20-25 minutes until crispy.

4. In a large bowl, combine romaine lettuce, cherry tomatoes, and vegan Caesar dressing.

5. Top with chickpea croutons and sprinkle with nutritional yeast.

Mediterranean Hummus Wrap

Ingredients:

- 4 whole wheat wraps or tortillas
- 1 cup hummus
- 2 cups mixed greens
- 1 cup cucumber, thinly sliced
- 1/2 cup cherry tomatoes, halved
- 1/4 cup red onion, thinly sliced
- 1/4 cup Kalamata olives, pitted and sliced
- 1/4 cup fresh parsley, chopped
- Juice of 1 lemon
- Salt and pepper to taste

Instructions:

1. Lay out the wraps and spread a generous layer of hummus on each.

2. Layer mixed greens, cucumber, cherry tomatoes, red onion, and Kalamata olives on top.

3. Sprinkle with fresh parsley and drizzle with lemon juice.

4. Season with salt and pepper.

5. Roll up the wraps, slice in half, and serve.

Roasted Vegetable and Quinoa Bowl

Ingredients:

- 1 cup quinoa, rinsed
- 2 cups vegetable broth
- 2 cups mixed vegetables (e.g., bell peppers, zucchini, carrots)
- 2 tablespoons olive oil
- 1 teaspoon dried herbs (e.g., thyme, rosemary)
- Salt and pepper to taste
- Balsamic vinaigrette dressing

Instructions:

1. Preheat your oven to 400°F (200°C).

2. Toss mixed vegetables with olive oil, dried herbs, salt, and pepper.

3. Roast vegetables for 20-25 minutes or until tender and slightly caramelized.

4. In a saucepan, cook quinoa in vegetable broth according to package instructions.

5. Assemble quinoa and roasted vegetables in bowls.

6. Drizzle with balsamic vinaigrette dressing before serving.

Vegan Eggplant Parmesan

Ingredients:

- 2 large eggplants, sliced into rounds
- 1 cup vegan breadcrumbs
- 1 cup marinara sauce
- 1 cup vegan mozzarella cheese, shredded
- 1/4 cup fresh basil leaves
- Olive oil for frying
- Salt and pepper to taste

Instructions:

1. Preheat your oven to 375°F (190°C).

2. Heat olive oil in a pan over medium heat.

3. Dredge eggplant slices in breadcrumbs, then fry until golden brown.

4. In a baking dish, layer marinara sauce, fried eggplant slices, and vegan mozzarella cheese.

5. Repeat layers until all ingredients are used, finishing with a layer of cheese on top.

6. Bake for 25-30 minutes or until bubbly and cheese is melted.

7. Garnish with fresh basil leaves before serving.

Sweet Potato and Black Bean Tacos

Ingredients:

- 2 large sweet potatoes, peeled and cubed
- 1 can black beans, drained and rinsed
- 1 red onion, thinly sliced
- 1 teaspoon chili powder
- 1 teaspoon cumin
- 1/2 teaspoon paprika
- 1/4 cup fresh cilantro, chopped
- 8 small corn tortillas
- Salsa and avocado for topping

Instructions:

1. Preheat your oven to 400°F (200°C).

2. Toss sweet potato cubes with olive oil, chili powder, cumin, paprika, salt, and pepper.

3. Roast sweet potatoes for 20-25 minutes or until tender.

4. In a skillet, sauté red onion until softened.

5. Add black beans and cook until heated through.

6. Warm corn tortillas.

7. Assemble tacos with sweet potatoes, black bean mixture, salsa, avocado, and cilantro.

Vegan Greek Salad

Ingredients:

- 4 cups mixed greens
- 1 cucumber, diced
- 1 cup cherry tomatoes, halved
- 1/4 cup red onion, thinly sliced
- 1/4 cup Kalamata olives, pitted
- 1/4 cup vegan feta cheese, crumbled
- Fresh oregano leaves for garnish
- Greek dressing

Instructions:

1. In a large bowl, combine mixed greens, diced cucumber, cherry tomatoes, red onion, Kalamata olives, and vegan feta cheese.
2. Drizzle with Greek dressing and toss to coat.
3. Garnish with fresh oregano leaves before serving.

Curry Chickpea Salad

Ingredients:

-   2 cans chickpeas, drained and rinsed
-   1/2 cup celery, finely chopped
-   1/4 cup red onion, finely chopped
-   1/4 cup vegan mayonnaise
-   2 tablespoons curry powder
-   Juice of 1 lemon
-   Salt and pepper to taste
-   Fresh cilantro for garnish

Instructions:

1. In a large bowl, mash chickpeas with a fork or potato masher.

2. Add finely chopped celery, red onion, vegan mayonnaise, curry powder, lemon juice, salt, and pepper.

3. Mix until well combined.

4. Garnish with fresh cilantro before serving.

Chapter 4: Dinner Recipes

In this chapter, you'll discover an array of delectable dinner recipes designed to tantalize your taste buds while keeping your health in mind. These vegan creations are not only bursting with flavor but also tailored to meet the dietary needs of a diabetic kidney-friendly meal plan.

Vegan Lentil Shepherd's Pie

Ingredients:

- 1 cup dried green or brown lentils
- 4 cups vegetable broth
- 2 cups diced carrots
- 1 cup diced celery
- 1 cup diced onions
- 2 cloves garlic, minced
- 1 teaspoon dried thyme
- 1 teaspoon dried rosemary
- Salt and pepper to taste
- 4 cups mashed sweet potatoes

Instructions:

1. Cook lentils in vegetable broth until tender, about 25 minutes.
2. In a separate pan, sauté carrots, celery, onions, and garlic until tender.
3. Combine lentils, sautéed vegetables, thyme, rosemary, salt, and pepper in a baking dish.
4. Top with mashed sweet potatoes and bake at 350°F (175°C) until golden brown.

Zucchini Noodles with Pesto

Ingredients:

- 4 medium zucchinis, spiralized into noodles
- 1 cup fresh basil leaves
- 1/4 cup pine nuts
- 2 cloves garlic
- 1/4 cup nutritional yeast
- 1/4 cup olive oil
- Salt and pepper to taste
- Cherry tomatoes for garnish

Instructions:

1. In a blender, combine basil, pine nuts, garlic, nutritional yeast, olive oil, salt, and pepper to make pesto.

2. Toss zucchini noodles with pesto until well coated.

3. Garnish with cherry tomatoes and serve.

Butternut Squash Risotto

Ingredients:

*   2 cups diced butternut squash
*   1 1/2 cups Arborio rice
*   4 cups vegetable broth
*   1 cup diced onions
*   2 cloves garlic, minced
*   1/4 cup nutritional yeast
*   Salt and pepper to taste
*   Fresh sage leaves for garnish

Instructions:

1. Roast butternut squash until tender and set aside.

2. In a pan, sauté onions and garlic until translucent.

3. Add Arborio rice and cook for a few minutes.

4. Gradually add vegetable broth, stirring until absorbed.

5. Stir in roasted butternut squash, nutritional yeast, salt, and pepper.

6. Garnish with fresh sage leaves.

Vegan Chili

Ingredients:

- 2 cups cooked and drained kidney beans
- 2 cups cooked and drained black beans
- 1 cup diced onions
- 1 cup diced bell peppers
- 2 cloves garlic, minced
- 1 can (28 oz) crushed tomatoes
- 2 tablespoons chili powder
- 1 teaspoon cumin
- Salt and pepper to taste
- Fresh cilantro for garnish

Instructions:

1. In a pot, sauté onions, bell peppers, and garlic until soft.

2. Add crushed tomatoes, kidney beans, black beans, chili powder, cumin, salt, and pepper.

3. Simmer for 20-30 minutes.

4. Garnish with fresh cilantro.

Vegan Stuffed Cabbage Rolls

Ingredients:

- 8 large cabbage leaves
- 1 cup cooked brown rice
- 1 cup cooked lentils
- 1 cup diced tomatoes
- 1/2 cup diced onions
- 2 cloves garlic, minced
- 1 teaspoon paprika
- Salt and pepper to taste
- 1 can (14 oz) tomato sauce

Instructions:

1. Blanch cabbage leaves in boiling water for a few minutes until soft.

2. In a bowl, combine cooked brown rice, lentils, diced tomatoes, onions, garlic, paprika, salt, and pepper.

3. Place a spoonful of the mixture onto each cabbage leaf and roll them up.

4. Arrange the rolls in a baking dish and top with tomato sauce.

5. Bake at 350°F (175°C) for about 30 minutes.

Portobello Mushroom Steaks

Ingredients:

- 4 large portobello mushrooms
- 1/4 cup balsamic vinegar
- 2 tablespoons olive oil
- 2 cloves garlic, minced
- 1 teaspoon dried thyme
- Salt and pepper to taste

Instructions:

1. In a bowl, mix balsamic vinegar, olive oil, garlic, thyme, salt, and pepper.

2. Marinate portobello mushrooms in the mixture for 20-30 minutes.

3. Grill or roast the mushrooms until tender, about 10 minutes per side.

Cauliflower and Chickpea Curry

Ingredients:

- 1 medium cauliflower, cut into florets
- 2 cups cooked chickpeas
- 1 cup diced onions
- 2 cloves garlic, minced
- 1 can (14 oz) diced tomatoes
- 1 can (14 oz) coconut milk
- 2 tablespoons curry powder
- Salt and pepper to taste
- Fresh cilantro for garnish

Instructions:

1. In a pan, sauté onions and garlic until translucent.
2. Add cauliflower florets, cooked chickpeas, diced tomatoes, coconut milk, curry powder, salt, and pepper.
3. Simmer until cauliflower is tender, about 15-20 minutes.
4. Garnish with fresh cilantro.

Vegan Jambalaya

Ingredients:

- 1 cup brown rice
- 1 cup diced bell peppers
- 1 cup diced celery
- 1 cup diced onions
- 1 cup diced tomatoes
- 2 cloves garlic, minced
- 1 teaspoon Cajun seasoning
- 1/2 teaspoon paprika
- Salt and pepper to taste

Instructions:

1. Cook brown rice according to package instructions.
2. In a large skillet, sauté bell peppers, celery, onions, and garlic until softened.
3. Add cooked rice, diced tomatoes, Cajun seasoning, paprika, salt, and pepper.
4. Cook for an additional 10 minutes.

Spinach and Artichoke Stuffed Peppers

Ingredients:

- 4 large bell peppers, halved and seeded
- 2 cups fresh spinach, chopped
- 1 cup canned artichoke hearts, chopped
- 1 cup cooked quinoa
- 1/2 cup diced onions
- 2 cloves garlic, minced
- 1/4 cup nutritional yeast
- Salt and pepper to taste

Instructions:

1. Steam bell peppers until slightly tender, about 5 minutes. Set aside.
2. In a skillet, sauté onions and garlic until translucent.
3. Combine spinach, artichoke hearts, quinoa, nutritional yeast, sautéed onions, garlic, salt, and pepper in a bowl.
4. Stuff the bell peppers with the mixture.
5. Bake at 375°F (190°C) for 20-25 minutes.

Vegan Pad Thai

Ingredients:

- 8 oz rice noodles
- 1 cup diced tofu
- 1 cup bean sprouts
- 1/2 cup chopped peanuts
- 2 cloves garlic, minced
- 1/4 cup soy sauce
- 2 tablespoons tamarind paste
- 2 tablespoons maple syrup
- Juice of 1 lime
- Chili flakes (optional)
- Fresh cilantro for garnish

Instructions:

1. Cook rice noodles according to package instructions.
2. In a pan, sauté tofu and garlic until tofu is lightly browned.
3. Add cooked rice noodles, bean sprouts, chopped peanuts, soy sauce, tamarind paste, maple syrup, lime juice, and chili flakes (if desired).

4. Toss and cook for a few minutes until heated through.

5. Garnish with fresh cilantro.

Creamy Vegan Mushroom Pasta

Ingredients:

- 8 oz whole wheat pasta
- 2 cups sliced mushrooms
- 1 cup diced onions
- 2 cloves garlic, minced
- 1 cup unsweetened almond milk
- 2 tablespoons nutritional yeast
- 1 tablespoon olive oil
- Salt and pepper to taste
- Fresh parsley for garnish

Instructions:

1. Cook pasta according to package instructions.
2. In a skillet, sauté mushrooms, onions, and garlic until tender.

3. Add almond milk, nutritional yeast, olive oil, salt, and pepper. Cook until the sauce thickens.

4. Toss the cooked pasta in the creamy mushroom sauce.

5. Garnish with fresh parsley.

Vegan BBQ Tofu Skewers

Ingredients:

- 1 block extra-firm tofu, cubed
- 1 cup BBQ sauce (check for sugar content)
- 1 bell pepper, cut into chunks
- 1 red onion, cut into chunks
- Wooden skewers, soaked in water

Instructions:

1. Marinate tofu cubes in BBQ sauce for at least 30 minutes.

2. Thread tofu, bell pepper, and red onion onto the soaked skewers.

3. Grill or broil until tofu is lightly charred and vegetables are tender, basting with more BBQ sauce as needed.

Vegan Eggplant and Tomato Bake

Ingredients:

- 2 large eggplants, sliced

- 2 cups diced tomatoes

- 1 cup diced onions

- 2 cloves garlic, minced

- 1/4 cup chopped fresh basil

- 1/4 cup olive oil

- Salt and pepper to taste

- Vegan mozzarella cheese (optional)

Instructions:

1. Preheat the oven to 375°F (190°C).

2. In a baking dish, layer sliced eggplants, diced tomatoes, onions, and minced garlic.

3. Drizzle olive oil over the layers and season with salt and pepper.

4. Repeat the layers.

5. Bake for 30-40 minutes until eggplants are tender.

6. If desired, sprinkle with vegan mozzarella cheese and bake for an additional 10 minutes until bubbly.

Vegan Spaghetti Carbonara

Ingredients:

- 8 oz whole wheat spaghetti
- 1 cup frozen green peas
- 1 cup diced vegan bacon or tempeh
- 2 cloves garlic, minced
- 1/2 cup unsweetened almond milk
- 1/4 cup nutritional yeast
- Salt and pepper to taste
- Fresh parsley for garnish

Instructions:

1. Cook spaghetti according to package instructions, adding frozen peas in the last 3 minutes.
2. In a skillet, sauté vegan bacon or tempeh and garlic until crispy.
3. Combine cooked spaghetti, peas, sautéed vegan bacon, almond milk, nutritional yeast, salt, and pepper.
4. Cook for a few minutes until heated through.
5. Garnish with fresh parsley.

Quinoa-Stuffed Acorn Squash

Ingredients:

- 2 acorn squashes, halved and seeded
- 1 cup quinoa, cooked
- 1 cup diced apples
- 1/2 cup dried cranberries
- 1/4 cup chopped pecans
- 1 tablespoon maple syrup
- 1 teaspoon cinnamon
- Salt and pepper to taste

Instructions:

1. Roast acorn squashes until tender, about 30-40 minutes.
2. In a bowl, mix cooked quinoa, diced apples, dried cranberries, chopped pecans, maple syrup, cinnamon, salt, and pepper.
3. Stuff the roasted acorn squashes with the quinoa mixture.
4. Serve warm.

Chapter 5: Snacks and Appetizers

In this chapter, we dive into the world of delectable snacks and appetizers that are not only vegan but also incredibly satisfying. Whether you're hosting a gathering or simply craving a midday nibble, these recipes are sure to please your taste buds.

Guacamole with Veggie Sticks

Ingredients:

- 3 ripe avocados
- 1 small red onion, finely diced
- 2 tomatoes, diced
- 1-2 cloves garlic, minced
- Juice of 2 limes
- Salt and pepper to taste
- Assorted veggie sticks (carrots, celery, bell peppers) for dipping

Instructions:

1. Cut the avocados in half, remove the pits, and scoop the flesh into a bowl.

2. Mash the avocados with a fork until creamy but slightly chunky.

3. Add the diced onion, tomatoes, minced garlic, and lime juice. Mix well.

4. Season with salt and pepper to taste.

5. Serve the guacamole with an array of colorful veggie sticks for dipping.

Vegan Spinach and Artichoke Dip

Ingredients:

- 1 cup cooked spinach, drained and chopped
- 1 cup canned artichoke hearts, drained and chopped
- 1 cup vegan cream cheese
- 1/2 cup vegan mayonnaise
- 1/2 cup nutritional yeast
- 1/4 cup diced red bell pepper
- 1/4 cup diced onion
- 2 cloves garlic, minced
- Salt and pepper to taste

- Tortilla chips for dipping

Instructions:

1. In a mixing bowl, combine the vegan cream cheese, vegan mayonnaise, and nutritional yeast.
2. Stir in the chopped spinach, artichoke hearts, red bell pepper, onion, and minced garlic.
3. Season with salt and pepper to taste.
4. Transfer the mixture to a baking dish and bake at 350°F (175°C) for 20-25 minutes, or until bubbly and lightly golden.
5. Serve the vegan spinach and artichoke dip with tortilla chips for a creamy, savory treat.

Roasted Chickpeas

Ingredients:

- 2 cans (15 ounces each) chickpeas, drained and rinsed
- 2 tablespoons olive oil
- 1 teaspoon paprika
- 1/2 teaspoon cumin
- 1/2 teaspoon garlic powder

- Salt and pepper to taste

Instructions:

1. Preheat your oven to 400°F (200°C).

2. In a bowl, toss the chickpeas with olive oil, paprika, cumin, garlic powder, salt, and pepper.

3. Spread the seasoned chickpeas on a baking sheet in a single layer.

4. Roast for 25-30 minutes, or until crispy and golden.

5. Allow them to cool slightly before serving as a crunchy and protein-packed snack.

Vegan Salsa and Tortilla Chips

Ingredients:

- 2 cups diced tomatoes
- 1/2 cup diced red onion
- 1/4 cup chopped cilantro
- Juice of 1 lime
- Salt and pepper to taste
- Tortilla chips for dipping

Instructions:

1. In a bowl, combine the diced tomatoes, red onion, cilantro, and lime juice.
2. Season with salt and pepper to taste.
3. Serve the fresh vegan salsa with a side of tortilla chips for a zesty and satisfying snack.

Hummus and Cucumber Slices

Ingredients:

- 1 cup canned chickpeas, drained and rinsed
- 1/4 cup tahini
- Juice of 1 lemon
- 2 cloves garlic, minced
- 2 tablespoons olive oil
- 1/2 teaspoon ground cumin
- Salt and pepper to taste
- Cucumber slices for dipping

Instructions:

1. In a food processor, combine the chickpeas, tahini, lemon juice, minced garlic, olive oil, ground cumin, salt, and pepper.

2. Blend until smooth and creamy, adding a splash of water if needed to reach your desired consistency.

3. Transfer the hummus to a serving bowl and drizzle with a bit of olive oil.

4. Serve with fresh cucumber slices for a refreshing and nutritious dip.

Vegan Caprese Skewers

Ingredients:

- Cherry tomatoes
- Fresh basil leaves
- Vegan mozzarella-style cheese, cubed
- Balsamic glaze (store-bought or homemade)
- Wooden skewers

Instructions:

1. Thread a cherry tomato, a basil leaf, and a cube of vegan mozzarella onto each wooden skewer.

2. Arrange the skewers on a serving platter.

3. Drizzle with balsamic glaze for a sweet and tangy finish.

Edamame with Sea Salt

Ingredients:

- 2 cups frozen edamame (in pods)
- Sea salt to taste

Instructions:

1. Cook the frozen edamame according to the package instructions.
2. Drain and pat them dry.
3. Sprinkle with sea salt and serve as a simple and protein-rich snack.

Vegan Buffalo Cauliflower Bites

Ingredients:

- 1 head cauliflower, cut into florets
- 1 cup vegan buffalo sauce
- 1 cup almond flour
- 1 cup water
- 1 teaspoon garlic powder
- 1 teaspoon paprika
- Salt and pepper to taste

- Vegan ranch or blue cheese dressing for dipping (optional)

Instructions:

1. Preheat your oven to 450°F (230°C).
2. In a bowl, whisk together the almond flour, water, garlic powder, paprika, salt, and pepper to create a batter.
3. Dip each cauliflower floret into the batter, ensuring it's well coated, and place them on a baking sheet lined with parchment paper.
4. Bake for 20-25 minutes or until the cauliflower is crispy and golden.
5. Toss the baked cauliflower in the vegan buffalo sauce until evenly coated.
6. Serve with vegan ranch or blue cheese dressing if desired for a spicy and satisfying snack.

Stuffed Mushrooms

Ingredients:

- 15 large mushrooms, cleaned and stems removed
- 1 cup vegan cream cheese

- 1/4 cup breadcrumbs
- 2 cloves garlic, minced
- 2 tablespoons chopped fresh parsley
- Salt and pepper to taste

Instructions:

1. Preheat your oven to 375°F (190°C).
2. In a bowl, mix the vegan cream cheese, breadcrumbs, minced garlic, chopped parsley, salt, and pepper until well combined.
3. Stuff each mushroom cap with the cream cheese mixture.
4. Place the stuffed mushrooms on a baking sheet and bake for 15-20 minutes, or until the tops are golden and the mushrooms are tender.
5. Serve these delightful stuffed mushrooms as a flavorful appetizer.

Vegan Spring Rolls

Ingredients:

- Rice paper wrappers

- Assorted veggies (e.g., carrots, cucumbers, bell peppers, lettuce)
- Fresh herbs (e.g., mint, basil)
- Cooked rice vermicelli noodles (optional)
- Peanut dipping sauce (store-bought or homemade)

Instructions:

1. Dip a rice paper wrapper in warm water for a few seconds until it softens.
2. Lay it flat on a clean surface.
3. Layer your choice of veggies, herbs, and rice vermicelli noodles (if using) in the center.
4. Fold the sides in and roll it up tightly, similar to a burrito.
5. Serve with a flavorful peanut dipping sauce for a light and refreshing appetizer.

Vegan Bruschetta

Ingredients:

- Baguette or crusty bread slices
- Ripe tomatoes, diced
- Fresh basil leaves, chopped

- Garlic cloves, minced

- Extra virgin olive oil

- Balsamic vinegar

- Salt and pepper to taste

Instructions:

1. Toast the bread slices until they are slightly crispy.

2. In a bowl, combine the diced tomatoes, chopped basil, minced garlic, a drizzle of olive oil, a splash of balsamic vinegar, salt, and pepper.

3. Spoon the tomato mixture onto the toasted bread slices.

4. Serve as a classic and flavorful Italian appetizer.

Vegan Popcorn with Nutritional Yeast

Ingredients:

- 1/2 cup popcorn kernels

- 2 tablespoons nutritional yeast

- 2 tablespoons vegan butter

- Salt to taste

Instructions:

1. Pop the popcorn kernels using your preferred method (stove, microwave, or popcorn maker).
2. Melt the vegan butter in a small saucepan.
3. Drizzle the melted butter over the popped popcorn, tossing to coat evenly.
4. Sprinkle nutritional yeast and a pinch of salt over the popcorn and toss again.
5. Serve this savory and slightly cheesy vegan popcorn as a guilt-free snack during movie night.

Vegan Sweet Potato Fries

Ingredients:

- 2 large sweet potatoes, cut into fries
- 2 tablespoons olive oil
- 1 teaspoon paprika
- 1/2 teaspoon garlic powder
- Salt and pepper to taste

Instructions:

1. Preheat your oven to 425°F (220°C).

2. In a bowl, toss the sweet potato fries with olive oil, paprika, garlic powder, salt, and pepper.

3. Spread the fries in a single layer on a baking sheet.

4. Bake for 25-30 minutes, flipping them halfway through, until they are crispy and golden.

5. Serve these sweet and savory fries as a delightful side or snack.

Vegan Olive Tapenade

Ingredients:

- 1 cup pitted black olives
- 1/4 cup capers
- 2 cloves garlic
- 2 tablespoons fresh lemon juice
- 2 tablespoons extra virgin olive oil
- Freshly ground black pepper to taste
- Toasted baguette slices or crackers for serving

Instructions:

1. In a food processor, combine the black olives, capers, garlic, lemon juice, and olive oil.

2. Pulse until the mixture is coarsely chopped and well combined.

3. Season with freshly ground black pepper to taste.

4. Serve this zesty vegan olive tapenade with toasted baguette slices or crackers for a flavorful appetizer.

Vegan Nachos with Cashew Cheese

Ingredients:

- Tortilla chips
- 1 cup cashews, soaked and drained
- 1/4 cup nutritional yeast
- 1/4 cup water
- Juice of 1 lime
- 1 teaspoon cumin
- 1/2 teaspoon chili powder
- Salt to taste
- Sliced jalapeños, black beans, diced tomatoes, and chopped cilantro for topping

Instructions:

1. In a blender, combine the soaked cashews, nutritional yeast, water, lime juice, cumin, chili powder, and salt.
2. Blend until you have a creamy cashew cheese sauce.
3. Arrange a layer of tortilla chips on a serving platter.
4. Drizzle the cashew cheese sauce over the chips.
5. Top with sliced jalapeños, black beans, diced tomatoes, and chopped cilantro.
6. Serve these loaded vegan nachos as a crowd-pleasing snack or appetizer.

Chapter 6: Desserts

In Chapter 6, we dive into the world of delectable vegan desserts, proving that a plant-based diet can satisfy your sweet cravings just as well as any other. These recipes not only tantalize your taste buds but also keep in mind your health, making them suitable for a diabetic-friendly lifestyle.

Vegan Chocolate Avocado Mousse

Ingredients:

- 2 ripe avocados
- 1/4 cup cocoa powder
- 1/4 cup maple syrup
- 1 tsp vanilla extract
- A pinch of salt

Instructions:

1. Blend avocados until creamy.
2. Add cocoa powder, maple syrup, vanilla, and salt.
3. Blend until smooth and refrigerate before serving.

Vegan Blueberry Crisp

Ingredients:

- 4 cups fresh blueberries
- 1 cup rolled oats
- 1/2 cup almond flour
- 1/4 cup maple syrup
- 2 tbsp coconut oil
- A pinch of cinnamon

Instructions:

1. Mix blueberries with maple syrup and spread in a baking dish.
2. Combine oats, almond flour, coconut oil, and cinnamon. Crumble over blueberries.
3. Bake at 350°F (175°C) for 30 minutes.

Vegan Banana Ice Cream

Ingredients:

- 4 ripe bananas, frozen
- 1/4 cup almond milk
- 1 tsp vanilla extract

Instructions:

1. Blend frozen bananas, almond milk, and vanilla until creamy.
2. Freeze for an hour for a firmer texture.

Almond and Raspberry Thumbprint Cookies

Ingredients:

-   1 cup almond meal
-   1/4 cup maple syrup
-   1/4 cup raspberry jam

Instructions:

1. Combine almond meal and maple syrup.
2. Form small balls, press thumb in the center, and add raspberry jam.
3. Bake at 350°F (175°C) for 10-12 minutes.

Vegan Rice Pudding

Ingredients:

-   1 cup cooked rice

- 2 cups almond milk
- 1/4 cup maple syrup
- 1 tsp vanilla extract
- A pinch of cinnamon

Instructions:

1. Combine rice, almond milk, maple syrup, and vanilla in a pot.
2. Simmer, stirring often, until thick.
3. Sprinkle with cinnamon before serving.

Vegan Chocolate Chip Cookies

Ingredients:

- 2 cups almond flour
- 1/2 cup maple syrup
- 1/4 cup coconut oil
- 1/2 cup vegan chocolate chips

Instructions:

1. Mix almond flour, maple syrup, and coconut oil.
2. Fold in chocolate chips.
3. Bake at 350°F (175°C) for 12-15 minutes.

Vegan Apple Crumble

Ingredients:

- 4 cups sliced apples
- 1 cup rolled oats
- 1/4 cup almond flour
- 1/4 cup maple syrup
- 2 tbsp coconut oil
- A pinch of nutmeg

Instructions:

1. Mix apples with nutmeg and spread in a baking dish.
2. Combine oats, almond flour, maple syrup, and coconut oil. Crumble over apples.
3. Bake at 350°F (175°C) for 30 minutes.

Vegan Lemon Bars

Ingredients:

- 1 cup almond flour
- 1/4 cup maple syrup
- 1/4 cup lemon juice
- Zest of 1 lemon

Instructions:

1. Mix almond flour, maple syrup, lemon juice, and lemon zest.
2. Press into a pan and bake at 350°F (175°C) for 20 minutes.
3. Let cool before slicing.

Vegan Chocolate Pots de Crème

Ingredients:

- 1 cup coconut milk
- 1/4 cup cocoa powder
- 1/4 cup maple syrup
- 1 tsp vanilla extract

Instructions:

1. Heat coconut milk, cocoa powder, and maple syrup in a pot until hot but not boiling.
2. Remove from heat, stir in vanilla, and pour into ramekins.
3. Chill in the fridge until set.

Vegan Pumpkin Pie

Ingredients:

- 1 1/2 cups pumpkin puree
- 1/2 cup almond milk
- 1/4 cup maple syrup
- 1 tsp cinnamon
- 1/2 tsp nutmeg

Instructions:

1. Mix pumpkin puree, almond milk, maple syrup, cinnamon, and nutmeg.
2. Pour into a pie crust and bake at 350°F (175°C) for 40-45 minutes.

Vegan Berry Sorbet

Ingredients:

- 2 cups mixed berries (frozen)
- 1/4 cup maple syrup
- Juice of 1/2 lemon

Instructions:

1. Blend berries, maple syrup, and lemon juice until smooth.
2. Freeze for a few hours, stirring occasionally.

Vegan Peanut Butter Cups

Ingredients:

*   1/2 cup vegan chocolate chips
*   1/4 cup peanut butter

Instructions:

1. Melt chocolate chips in a microwave or on the stove.
2. Line a muffin tin with paper liners. Pour a little chocolate into each.
3. Add a spoonful of peanut butter and cover with more chocolate.
4. Freeze until solid.

Vegan Tiramisu

Ingredients:

*   1 cup brewed coffee, cooled

- 1/2 cup coconut cream

- 1/4 cup maple syrup

- 1 tsp cocoa powder

Instructions:

1. Dip vegan ladyfingers in coffee and place in a dish.

2. Whisk coconut cream and maple syrup until creamy.

3. Spread over the ladyfingers and dust with cocoa powder.

4. Refrigerate for a few hours.

Vegan Coconut Macaroons

Ingredients:

- 2 cups shredded coconut

- 1/4 cup maple syrup

- 1/4 cup coconut oil

Instructions:

1. Mix shredded coconut, maple syrup, and melted coconut oil.

2. Form into small macaroons and bake at 350°F (175°C) for 10-12 minutes.

Vegan Carrot Cake

Ingredients:

- 2 cups grated carrots
- 1 cup almond flour
- 1/4 cup maple syrup
- 1 tsp cinnamon
- 1/2 tsp nutmeg

Instructions:

1. Combine grated carrots, almond flour, maple syrup, cinnamon, and nutmeg.
2. Press into a cake pan and bake at 350°F (175°C) for 25-30 minutes.

Chapter 7: Smoothies

These smoothies are not just delicious; they are packed with essential nutrients, antioxidants, and fiber to keep you energized throughout the day. Whether you're looking for a morning boost or a post-workout recovery, these smoothie recipes have got you covered.

Green Detox Smoothie

Ingredients:

- 1 cup fresh spinach leaves
- 1/2 cucumber, peeled and sliced
- 1/2 green apple, cored and chopped
- 1/2 lemon, juiced
- 1 cup water or coconut water
- Ice cubes (optional)

Instructions:

1. Place all ingredients in a blender.
2. Blend until smooth and creamy.
3. Add ice cubes if desired, and blend again.

Vegan Berry Blast Smoothie

Ingredients:

- 1 cup mixed berries (strawberries, blueberries, raspberries)
- 1/2 banana
- 1 cup almond milk
- 1 tablespoon chia seeds
- 1 teaspoon honey or maple syrup (optional)

Instructions:

1. Combine all ingredients in a blender.
2. Blend until the mixture is smooth and the chia seeds are well incorporated.
3. Sweeten with honey or maple syrup if desired.

Chocolate Almond Butter Smoothie

Ingredients:

- 2 tablespoons almond butter
- 2 tablespoons cocoa powder
- 1 banana
- 1 cup almond milk

- 1 tablespoon honey or agave syrup (optional)

Instructions:

1. Place almond butter, cocoa powder, banana, and almond milk in a blender.
2. Blend until the mixture is creamy and smooth.
3. Sweeten with honey or agave syrup if desired.

Vegan Tropical Paradise Smoothie

Ingredients:

- 1/2 cup frozen pineapple chunks
- 1/2 cup frozen mango chunks
- 1/2 banana
- 1 cup coconut milk
- 1/4 cup orange juice

Instructions:

1. Combine all ingredients in a blender.
2. Blend until smooth and creamy.

Vegan Spinach and Pineapple Smoothie

Ingredients:

- 2 cups fresh spinach leaves
- 1 cup frozen pineapple chunks
- 1/2 banana
- 1 cup coconut water

Instructions:

1. Place spinach, pineapple, banana, and coconut water in a blender.
2. Blend until the mixture is smooth and vibrant green.

Blueberry and Kale Power Smoothie

Ingredients:

- 1 cup kale leaves, stems removed
- 1 cup frozen blueberries
- 1/2 banana
- 1 cup almond milk
- 1 tablespoon flaxseeds

Instructions:

1. Combine kale, blueberries, banana, almond milk, and flaxseeds in a blender.
2. Blend until smooth and packed with nutrients.

Vegan Mango Tango Smoothie

Ingredients:

- 1 cup frozen mango chunks
- 1/2 banana
- 1/2 cup orange juice
- 1/2 cup coconut milk

Instructions:

1. Place mango, banana, orange juice, and coconut milk in a blender.
2. Blend until smooth and tropical.

Vegan Peanut Butter and Banana Smoothie

Ingredients:

- 2 tablespoons peanut butter

- 1 banana

- 1 cup almond milk

- 1 tablespoon honey or agave syrup (optional)

Instructions:

1. Combine peanut butter, banana, almond milk in a blender.
2. Blend until creamy and indulgent.
3. Sweeten with honey or agave syrup if desired.

Vegan Coconut and Raspberry Smoothie

Ingredients:

- 1/2 cup frozen raspberries
- 1/2 cup frozen strawberries
- 1/2 banana
- 1 cup coconut milk

Instructions:

1. Place raspberries, strawberries, banana, and coconut milk in a blender.

2. Blend until smooth and bursting with berry flavor.

Vegan Cherry Almond Smoothie

Ingredients:

- 1 cup frozen cherries
- 1/4 cup almonds
- 1/2 banana
- 1 cup almond milk

Instructions:

1. Combine cherries, almonds, banana, and almond milk in a blender.
2. Blend until the mixture is creamy and rich in cherry-almond goodness.

Vegan Espresso Protein Smoothie

Ingredients:

- 1 shot of espresso (cooled)
- 1/2 banana
- 1 cup almond milk
- 1 scoop vegan protein powder

- 1 teaspoon cocoa powder

Instructions:

1. Combine espresso, banana, almond milk, vegan protein powder, and cocoa powder in a blender.
2. Blend until the mixture is smooth and caffeinated.

Vegan Peach and Oatmeal Smoothie

Ingredients:

- 1 cup frozen peaches
- 1/4 cup rolled oats
- 1/2 banana
- 1 cup almond milk
- 1 teaspoon honey or agave syrup (optional)

Instructions:

1. Place peaches, rolled oats, banana, almond milk in a blender.
2. Blend until smooth and satisfying.
3. Sweeten with honey or agave syrup if desired.

Vegan Strawberry Kiwi Smoothie

Ingredients:

- 1 cup frozen strawberries
- 2 kiwis, peeled and sliced
- 1/2 banana
- 1 cup coconut water

Instructions:

1. Combine strawberries, kiwis, banana, and coconut water in a blender.
2. Blend until the mixture is smooth and delightfully fruity.

Vegan Watermelon Cucumber Cooler

Ingredients:

- 2 cups fresh watermelon chunks
- 1/2 cucumber, peeled and sliced
- 1/2 lime, juiced
- 1 cup coconut water

Instructions:

1. Place watermelon, cucumber, lime juice, and coconut water in a blender.

2. Blend until refreshing and hydrating.

Vegan Orange Creamsicle Smoothie

Ingredients:

- 2 oranges, peeled and segmented
- 1/2 banana
- 1 cup almond milk
- 1 teaspoon vanilla extract

Instructions:

1. Combine oranges, banana, almond milk, and vanilla extract in a blender.

2. Blend until smooth and reminiscent of a classic creamsicle.

CONCLUSION

As we come to the end of this journey through a vegan diabetic kidney diet meal plan, it's important to reflect on the valuable lessons we've learned and the positive changes we've made in our lives.

In this concluding chapter, we don't simply bid farewell; we open the door to a sustainable and health-conscious future. The choices we've made over the course of this meal plan aren't just short-term fixes; they are the building blocks of a healthier and happier existence.

Our culinary adventures have demonstrated that delicious and satisfying meals can be crafted from plant-based ingredients, even when navigating the complex terrain of diabetic kidney disease. We've learned the art of balancing flavors and textures, creating dishes that tantalize the taste buds while nourishing our bodies.

But it doesn't end here. The journey towards better health and well-being continues. It's a journey that extends far beyond the pages of this meal plan. The principles and recipes you've discovered here are your foundation, a springboard from which you can explore and experiment, crafting your own unique dishes and meal plans tailored to your tastes and dietary needs.

Remember, health is not a destination but a lifelong pursuit. Continue to make mindful choices, savor the joys of cooking and sharing meals, and seek out support and resources as you need them. Your path to better health is a personal one, and every step you take brings you closer to your goals.

So, as we close this chapter, let it be the beginning of a new chapter in your life—a chapter filled with vibrant health, delicious food, and the knowledge that you have the power to shape your well-being. Thank you for embarking on this journey with us, and may your future be filled with good health, happiness, and the joy of nourishing both body and soul.

www.ingramcontent.com/pod-product-compliance
Lightning Source LLC
Chambersburg PA
CBHW070825260726
48660CB00005B/1995